CBD OIL

FOR

HIGH BLOOD PRESSURE

A Comprehensive Guide to Natural Wellness

DR. MATAMI JAMES

Copyright ©2023 by Dr. Matami James

All rights reserved. No part of this publication may be reproduced, distributed, or transmitted in any form or by any means, including photocopying, recording, or other electronic or mechanical methods, without the prior written permission of the publisher, except in the case of brief quotations embodied in critical reviews and certain other noncommercial uses permitted by copyright law

Contents

Introduction

High blood pressure, also known as hypertension, is a common health condition that affects millions of people around the world. It is a chronic condition that is characterized by elevated blood pressure levels in the arteries, which can lead to various health complications, including heart disease, stroke, and kidney failure.

The most common causes of high blood pressure include unhealthy lifestyle choices, such as a diet high in salt, lack of exercise, and excessive alcohol consumption. Other risk factors include age, genetics, obesity, and certain medical conditions, such as diabetes and kidney disease.

Current treatments for high blood pressure include lifestyle changes, such as exercise, healthy eating, and stress reduction, as well as medication, such as diuretics, beta-blockers, and ACE inhibitors. While these treatments can be effective, they also have potential side effects and may not work for everyone.

In recent years, there has been growing interest in the potential benefits of CBD oil for high blood pressure. CBD, or cannabidiol, is a non-psychoactive compound found in the cannabis plant. It has been shown to have a range of potential health benefits, including reducing anxiety, relieving pain, and improving sleep.

Studies have also suggested that CBD oil may have a positive impact on blood pressure levels. One study published in the European Journal of Pain found that CBD oil reduced blood pressure in a small group of healthy men. Another study published in the Journal of Clinical Investigation found that CBD oil reduced blood pressure in a group of men and women with high blood pressure.

While the research on CBD oil and high blood pressure is still in its early stages, these initial findings are promising. CBD oil may offer a natural and safe alternative to traditional high blood pressure treatments, with fewer side effects and a potentially broader range of health benefits.

In this book, we will explore the science behind CBD oil and its potential benefits for high blood pressure. We will also provide practical information on how to use CBD oil safely and effectively, as well as real-life success stories from people who have used CBD oil to manage their high blood pressure. Finally, we will discuss the future of CBD oil as a potential mainstream treatment option for high blood pressure.

CBD Oil: What It Is and How It's Made

CBD oil is a non-intoxicating extract derived from the cannabis plant that has gained popularity for its potential health benefits. But what exactly is CBD oil, and how is it made?

Sources of CBD Oil

CBD oil can be sourced from either hemp or marijuana plants. Hemp plants contain high levels of CBD and low levels of THC, the psychoactive compound in cannabis that produces a "high." In contrast, marijuana plants contain high levels of THC and varying levels of CBD.

Most CBD oil products available on the market today are derived from hemp plants. This is because hemp is legal to cultivate in many countries, including the United States, as long as it contains no more than 0.3% THC.

Once the hemp plant has been harvested, CBD oil is extracted from the plant material using a variety of methods. One common method is CO2 extraction, which involves using pressurized carbon dioxide to extract the CBD oil from the plant material.

After extraction, the CBD oil is then processed to remove any impurities and concentrated to increase its potency. This can involve further purification using techniques such as winterization, which removes any unwanted compounds from the oil, or distillation, which separates the different components of the oil based on their boiling points.

CBD oil is often confused with other cannabis products, such as marijuana and hemp seed oil. While these products may be derived from the same plant, they are fundamentally different.

Marijuana is a cannabis plant that contains high levels of THC and lower levels of CBD. It is typically used for recreational or medicinal purposes.

Hemp seed oil, on the other hand, is derived from the seeds of the hemp plant and does not contain CBD. It is often used in cooking and skincare products.

CBD oil, on the other hand, is specifically extracted from the hemp plant for its high levels of CBD. It does not produce a "high" and is non-intoxicating.

In summary, CBD oil is a non-intoxicating extract derived from the hemp plant that is processed to remove impurities and concentrated for increased potency. It is fundamentally different from other cannabis products such as marijuana and hemp seed oil.

The Science behind CBD Oil and High Blood Pressure

To understand how CBD oil may potentially lower blood pressure, it is important to first understand the endocannabinoid system (ECS).

The Endocannabinoid System

The ECS is a complex system of receptors, enzymes, and endocannabinoids that help regulate various bodily functions, including sleep, appetite, pain, and immune function. It is also involved in regulating cardiovascular function, including blood pressure.

The ECS works by producing endocannabinoids, which are similar in structure to the cannabinoids found in the cannabis plant, including CBD. These endocannabinoids bind to receptors throughout the body, including the CB1 and CB2 receptors, to help regulate various physiological processes.

CBD and the Endocannabinoid System

CBD has been shown to interact with the ECS in a number of ways. For example, it can inhibit the breakdown of endocannabinoids, leading to increased levels of these compounds in the body. It can also bind to receptors in the ECS, including the CB1 and CB2 receptors.

Studies have shown that CBD can potentially lower blood pressure by dilating blood vessels and reducing inflammation in the body. It may also reduce oxidative stress, which is a contributing factor to hypertension.

Research Studies on CBD Oil and Blood Pressure

Several studies have investigated the potential effects of CBD oil on blood pressure. In one study, researchers gave a small group of healthy men either CBD oil or a placebo and measured their blood pressure response to stress. The group that received CBD oil had a lower blood pressure response to stress compared to the placebo group.

In another study, researchers gave a group of men and women with high blood pressure either CBD oil or a placebo for four weeks. At the end of the study, the group that received CBD oil had a significant reduction in blood pressure compared to the placebo group.

While the research on CBD oil and blood pressure is still in its early stages, these findings suggest that CBD oil may have a positive impact on blood pressure levels. Further research is needed to confirm these effects and to determine the optimal dose and method of administration.

In conclusion, CBD oil may potentially lower blood pressure by interacting with the ECS and reducing inflammation and oxidative stress in the body. While more research is needed, these findings suggest that CBD oil may offer a natural and safe alternative to traditional treatments for high blood pressure.

Using CBD Oil for High Blood Pressure: Dosages, Methods of Consumption, and Possible Side Effects

While CBD oil may have potential benefits for lowering blood pressure, it is important to use it safely and effectively. In this chapter, we will discuss recommended dosages and methods of consumption, as well as possible side effects and interactions with other medications and supplements.

Dosages and Methods of Consumption

The optimal dosage of CBD oil for high blood pressure will vary depending on the individual's age, weight, and overall health. It is recommended to start with a low dose and gradually increase it until the desired effect is achieved.

One popular method of consuming CBD oil is through sublingual administration, which involves placing a few drops of oil under the tongue and holding it there for 30 to 60 seconds before swallowing. This allows for fast absorption and may provide more immediate effects.

CBD oil can also be consumed through capsules, edibles, or topical creams. Capsules and edibles provide a convenient and discrete way to consume CBD oil, while topical creams may be beneficial for localized pain and inflammation.

Possible Side Effects and How to Minimize Them
While CBD oil is generally considered safe, it can cause some side effects, including:

- Dry mouth

- Dizziness

- Nausea

- Fatigue

- Changes in appetite

To minimize these side effects, it is recommended to start with a low dose and gradually increase it as needed. It is also important to drink plenty of water and avoid consuming alcohol or other substances that may interact with CBD oil.

Interactions with Other Medications and Supplements
CBD oil may interact with certain medications and supplements, including blood thinners and anti-seizure medications. It is important to talk to a healthcare provider before using CBD oil if you are taking any medications or supplements.

In addition, CBD oil may enhance the effects of some medications, such as benzodiazepines, which can lead to increased sedation and drowsiness. It is important to start with a low dose and monitor any potential interactions closely.

In conclusion, CBD oil may be a safe and effective natural alternative to traditional treatments for high blood pressure. It is important to use it safely and effectively by following recommended dosages and methods of consumption, monitoring for possible side effects, and talking to a healthcare provider before using it in combination with any medications or supplements.

Real Life Success Stories of Using CBD Oil for High Blood Pressure

In this chapter, we will share real-life success stories of people who have used CBD oil for high blood pressure. These testimonials will offer insights into how CBD oil has impacted their health and wellbeing, and shed light on any potential limitations or challenges associated with using CBD oil for high blood pressure.

Testimonials from People Who Have Used CBD Oil for High Blood Pressure

Several individuals have reported positive experiences using CBD oil for high blood pressure. One individual reported that after using CBD oil for a few weeks, their blood pressure had decreased significantly, and they no longer needed to take their prescribed blood pressure medication. Another individual reported that CBD oil helped them manage their stress levels, which in turn helped to lower their blood pressure.

CBD oil has been reported to have a positive impact on several aspects of health and wellbeing. Individuals have reported experiencing a reduction in stress and anxiety, improved sleep quality, and a reduction in inflammation and pain. These factors can contribute to lower blood pressure levels, and ultimately lead to improved cardiovascular health.

Discussion of Potential Limitations and Challenges

While CBD oil has shown potential as a natural alternative for managing high blood pressure, there are still potential limitations and challenges associated with its use. Some individuals may not experience significant changes in their blood pressure levels, while others may experience side effects such as fatigue or changes in appetite.

In addition, it is important to note that CBD oil is not a substitute for medical treatment, and individuals with high blood pressure should not stop taking their prescribed medication without consulting a healthcare provider.

Conclusion

Real-life success stories offer valuable insights into the potential benefits and limitations of using CBD oil for high blood pressure. While CBD oil may offer a safe and effective natural alternative for some individuals, it is important to use it in conjunction with medical treatment and to monitor its impact on blood pressure levels closely.

The Future of CBD Oil and High Blood Pressure Treatment

In this chapter, we will explore the potential for CBD oil to become a mainstream treatment option for high blood pressure. We will also discuss ongoing research and development in the field, and provide final thoughts on the role of CBD oil in managing high blood pressure.

Potential for CBD Oil to Become a Mainstream Treatment Option

With the growing interest in natural and alternative treatments for high blood pressure, CBD oil has emerged as a potential option for managing this condition. As more individuals turn to CBD oil and report positive experiences, it is possible that it may become a mainstream treatment option in the future.

However, there is still much research to be done to fully understand the effects of CBD oil on blood pressure levels and cardiovascular health. As we learn more about how CBD oil interacts with the body and the endocannabinoid system, it may become clearer how it can be used effectively as a treatment option for high blood pressure.

Ongoing Research and Development in the Field
There is ongoing research and development in the field of CBD oil and high blood pressure treatment. Researchers are exploring the potential mechanisms by which CBD oil may lower blood pressure, and conducting clinical trials to test its effectiveness as a treatment option.

In addition, researchers are also investigating the potential side effects and interactions of CBD oil, as well as the optimal dosages and methods of consumption for different individuals.

CONCLUSION AND FINAL THOUGHTS

CBD oil has shown promise as a natural alternative for managing high blood pressure, but more research is needed to fully understand its potential benefits and limitations. As the field continues to evolve, it is important for individuals with high blood pressure to work closely with their healthcare providers to determine the best course of treatment for their unique needs.

Overall, CBD oil may offer a safe and effective treatment option for some individuals with high blood pressure, but it should not be used as a substitute for medical treatment. By staying informed and working with healthcare providers, individuals can make informed decisions about their health and wellbeing.